ECZEMA

SIMPLE TIPS FOR GETTING A GLOWING SKIN

DR. J. SIMON

Contents

INTRODUCTION

Another name for eczema is atopic dermatitis, which is a chronic, all-over skin condition characterized by redness, swelling, and itching. This specific type of dermatitis typically begins in early childhood and can persist until maturity, though it can affect people of all ages. Eczema is not contagious, and although its exact cause is unknown, immune system, environmental, and genetic factors are believed to be involved.

Typical eczema traits include:

1. Skin irritation:

Redness, swelling, and irritation are signs of eczema-induced skin inflammation.

2. Scratching:

Itching is one of eczema's main symptoms. There might be a strong urge to scratch, which could aggravate the skin even more.

3. Dry Skin Type:

Dry, sensitive skin is a common feature of eczema sufferers. It could feel like rough or scaly skin.

4. Rash and lesions:

Eczema can cause rashes to manifest as blisters, seeping lesions, or little, elevated pimples.

5. Regions That Are Usually Affected:

Eczema is a common skin condition that affects the cheeks, hands, elbows, knees, and backs of the knees.

6. Causes:

Eczema symptoms can worsen due to a number of factors known as triggers. These include temperature fluctuations, stress, allergens, exposure to potent chemicals, and particular irritants.

7. Chronic Features:

Eczema is a chronic condition that goes through flare-ups and remissions. Controlling and averting flare-ups is a crucial aspect of treating it.

8. Triad of Atopic Patients:

The atopic triad includes eczema along with allergic rhinitis, asthma, and atopic dermatitis. These other allergic reactions may be more common in people with eczema.

Despite the fact that eczema cannot be cured, there are several treatment options that aim to reduce inflammation, alleviate symptoms, and prevent flare-ups. Topical corticosteroids, moisturizers, immunomodulators, and antihistamines are a few examples. Furthermore, identifying and avoiding triggers can be crucial to managing the illness.

Dermatologists and other medical professionals should work closely with eczema sufferers to develop a personalized treatment plan. Better managing the condition and improving quality of life can also be achieved by treating the underlying causes of eczema, avoiding known triggers, and implementing good skincare habits.

CHAPTER ONE

Different Types of Eczema

Eczema, another name for atopic dermatitis, can take many different forms. All kinds could have different characteristics and affect different age groups. Here are some common eczema forms:

1. Asthmatic dermatitis:

Early childhood is often the onset period for atopic dermatitis, the most common type of eczema. It is associated with an allergy reaction history in the family, encompassing asthma and rhinitis. Among the symptoms are redness, irritation, and inflammation of the skin, particularly on the hands, knees, elbows, and face.

2. In contact dermatitis:

The skin can become irritated and develop contact dermatitis when it comes into contact with irritants or allergens. Chemical or detergent exposure is the most common cause of irritant contact dermatitis. Allergy to a specific material, such as metals, makeup, or specific plants, can cause allergic contact dermatitis.

3. Skin Conditions with Nummular Skin:

Nummular dermatitis is characterized by irritated skin patches that resemble coins or ovals. Adults are typically affected, and arid environments are where it is more common. These spots could get crusts or blisters and could hurt a lot.

4. Dermatitis dyshidrotic:

Dyshidrotic eczema causes small, uncomfortable blisters that primarily affect the hands and feet. The area around the blisters may be peeling, swollen, and red. One can develop this type of dermatitis due to allergies, stress, or exposure to certain metals.

5. Segmental dermatitis:

A person with seborrheic dermatitis has oily, scaly, red skin. It usually affects regions with a high density of sebaceous glands, such as the scalp, face, and chest, which can result in dandruff. In babies, it can manifest as cradle cap, and it can persist into adulthood.

6. Stains from dermatitis:

Stasis dermatitis, usually associated with poor circulation, primarily affects the lower legs. Skin irritation, redness, and discolouration occur when there is an interruption in the blood flow within the veins.

7. Diabetic neurodermitis:

The characteristic feature of neurodermatitis is thick, scaly patches of skin that develop from repeatedly scraping or scratching in response to an initial skin irritation. Usually, the neck, wrists, or ankles are affected.

8. id reaction, also known as autoeczematization:

The term "autoeczematization," or "the id reaction," refers to the eczematous reaction that occurs in one area of the body in response to an underlying skin condition or irritation. A rash that is distinct from the primary infection site manifests itself.

9. Food allergies causing eczema:

A person may develop allergic eczema if they are exposed to specific allergens, such as foods, medications, or airborne allergens. It could manifest as a red, swollen, and itchy rash that spreads widely.

A successful treatment plan requires identifying the precise type of eczema. In order to manage symptoms and prevent flare-ups, dermatologists and other medical specialists are qualified to make accurate diagnoses and recommend specialized treatments.

Causes and Motivators

Though its exact cause is unknown, atopic dermatitis, also referred to as eczema, is believed to result from a complex interaction of immune system, environmental, and genetic factors. Although eczema is inherited, certain factors may exacerbate symptoms or trigger flare-ups. Here are a few potential causes and triggers for eczema:

1. Molecular Biology:

Family history has a major influence on when eczema first appears. Atopic dermatitis, asthma, and allergic rhinitis run in families, and these conditions may raise an individual's risk of developing eczema.

2. Immune System Deficit:

Unusual immune responses can lead to eczema development. The immune system of a person with eczema may overreact to specific stimuli, resulting in inflammation and skin symptoms.

3. breakdown of the skin barrier:

Skin that has lost its capacity to protect itself from allergens, irritants, and the environment may be more susceptible. An irritated skin barrier increases inflammation by allowing allergens to enter and moisture to escape.

4. Aspects of the Environment:

Environmental factors have the potential to exacerbate or even cause eczema symptoms. These include:

Changes in the weather: Sweating can occur on hot, humid days, while dry, cold air can lead to dry skin.

Certain types of clothing, perfumes, strong detergents, and soaps are examples of irritants.

Allergens: Dust mites, mold, pollen, and pet dander are common allergens that can aggravate eczema symptoms.

5. Intenseness

Stress and anxiety can make eczema flare-ups or worsen pre-existing symptoms of the condition. Stress management strategies could decrease these impacts.

6. hormones:

Hormonal changes, particularly during puberty, pregnancy, and menstruation, can affect how severe eczema symptoms are.

7. Intolerances:

Food allergies, dust allergies, and contact allergies to metals or latex materials can all cause or worsen eczema symptoms.

8. microbe infections:

Fungal, bacterial, or viral skin infections can trigger flare-ups of eczema. Staphylococcus aureus and Herpes simplex virus are common infections.

9. Grasping and Pulling:

The eczema symptoms can worsen and the skin can get thicker and leathery if excessive rubbing or scratching is done.

10. Certain Foods:

Food allergies may not be the primary cause of eczema, but for some individuals, certain foods can exacerbate or intensify symptoms. Common triggers include dairy, eggs, gluten, and nuts.

The key to managing eczema is being aware of and avoiding certain triggers. Patients with eczema should work closely with physicians to develop customized regimens for maintaining healthy skin, changing lifestyle choices, and preventing flare-ups. Dermatologists can prescribe medication when necessary, make recommendations for suitable products, and give advice on skincare routines.

Signs and Causes of Concern

Numerous symptoms and indicators related to the skin can be caused by atopic dermatitis, commonly referred to as eczema. These symptoms may vary in intensity and come and go over time. Typical eczema symptoms and indicators include the following:

1. Eczema (itching):

Eczema is primarily diagnosed by severe itching. Because of the severe itching, there can be strong impulses to scratch the affected areas.

2. erythema, or flushing:

Redness or flushing of the skin are common symptoms of eczema. This redness is caused by increased blood flow to the affected areas and inflammation.

3. an inflammatory reaction

Eczema-induced skin inflammation causes discomfort and swelling. The affected areas may appear swollen or puffed.

4. Dry Skin Type:

Eczema has been related to dry, sensitive skin. On the affected area, there may be rough, scaly, or flaky skin.

5. Rash

A rash with distinctive patterns may be the first sign of eczema. There could be blisters, elevated bumps, or red or brownish-gray patches on the rash.

6. Seductive and Crisp:

Clear fluid may occasionally seep from the skin that is impacted by eczema. When this liquid dries, crusting may result.

7. Discoloration of the Skin:

Skin pigmentation changes can be brought on by persistent inflammation and scratching. The affected skin may change in tone from the surrounding skin.

8. Skin Thickened (Lichenification):

Skin that is repeatedly rubbed or scratched may become thicker and harder. Lichenification is the term for this condition, which can have leathery patches as an appearance.

9. Excoriations, or open sores:

Open sores, skin fractures, or minor cuts can result from persistent scratching. These places are prone to getting infected.

10. swells

Swollen skin can result from inflammation, particularly in regions with a high concentration of eczema.

11. Growing Worse as You Get Older:

Although eczema usually starts in childhood, it can also appear later in life or last into adulthood. The symptoms could evolve over time and go through phases of getting better or getting worse.

12. Dispersal on the Body:

Though it can affect any part of the body, eczema most commonly affects the face, hands, wrists, elbows, knees, and backs of the knees.

Remember that eczema is a chronic condition that flares up and then goes into remission. The symptoms may worsen as a result of triggers like allergens, irritants, stress, and external circumstances. Treatment plans, which frequently include skincare practices, moisturizers, topical corticosteroids, and lifestyle adjustments, are intended to relieve symptoms, lessen inflammation, and stop flare-ups. Eczema sufferers should consult medical professionals for advice on an accurate diagnosis and suitable course of treatment.

Assessment and Diagnosis

Healthcare practitioners, usually dermatologists or allergists, must perform a thorough examination in order to diagnose and assess eczema. The clinical assessment, medical history, and, in certain situations, extra testing are the main sources of the diagnosis. The following are the essential procedures for diagnosing and treating eczema:

1. Background in Health:

Medical professionals will inquire about the patient's past medical history, encompassing any family history of eczema, asthma, or allergy disorders. We'll talk in-depth about the onset of symptoms, the pattern of flare-ups, and possible triggers.

2. Evaluation of the Body:

To evaluate the appearance, distribution, and severity of eczema symptoms, a comprehensive physical examination of the skin is performed. The face, hands, elbows, knees, and other frequently afflicted areas of the body may be examined by medical professionals.

3. Assessment of the Symptoms:

We carefully assess symptoms like itching, redness, inflammation, dry skin, rash, and any accompanying oozing or crusting. The diagnosis is confirmed when certain patterns are present, such as the distinctive eczema rash.

4. Removal of All Other Terms and Conditions:

Physicians might rule out other skin disorders that could resemble eczema. Differential diagnosis may be required to rule out conditions like psoriasis, contact dermatitis, or fungal infections.

5. Tests for patches:

Patch testing may be used in cases of suspected contact dermatitis in order to pinpoint particular allergens or irritants that may be causing the symptoms of eczema.

6. Rarely, a skin biopsy

A skin biopsy might be done in specific situations where the diagnosis is not clear or when it is necessary to rule out other skin conditions. In order to examine the skin tissue under a microscope, a tiny sample must be taken.

7. Allergy Examination:

To find possible allergens that might be causing eczema symptoms, allergy testing—such as blood or skin prick tests—may be advised. Dust mites, food particles, pollen, and animal dander are examples of allergens.

8. Assessment of Triggers:

An important part of the examination is determining and assessing probable triggers for flare-ups of eczema. Assessing exposure to irritants, alterations in the surrounding environment, or stressors may be part of this.

9. Observing and Following Up:

Eczema sufferers need to see doctors for follow-up appointments and continuous monitoring after receiving a diagnosis. Monitoring the condition's progression, modifying treatment strategies, and addressing any new issues are all made easier with regular examinations.

Eczema is primarily diagnosed clinically, with particular symptoms and the skin's unique look being taken into consideration. Effective management and long-term care of eczema require a cooperative approach between medical practitioners and eczema sufferers. Individualized treatment programs are developed for each patient, and lifestyle changes are frequently advised to control symptoms and avoid flare-ups.

CHAPTER TWO

Therapies Techniques

The goals of treating atopic dermatitis, or eczema, are to lessen inflammation, ease symptoms, and stop flare-ups. The majority of the time, management techniques combine skincare routines, lifestyle adjustments, and occasionally pharmaceuticals. The strategy may change depending on the intensity of the symptoms and personal circumstances. The following are typical eczema treatment methods:

1. Skincare and hydrating products:

For those who have eczema, regular and appropriate skincare is essential. To keep skin hydrated, use gentle, fragrance-free cleansers and moisturizers. Skin barrier maintenance and prevention are assisted by moisturizers.

2. Localized Corticosteroids:

Topical corticosteroids are anti-inflammatory drugs that are administered topically to the afflicted area of skin. They assist in lowering inflammation and itching during flare-ups. Depending on the location and severity of the eczema, medical professionals will recommend the right strength.

3. Inhibitors of Calcineurin on the Skin:

Calcineurin inhibitors: tacrolimus and pimecrolimus are non-steroidal drugs that can be used to treat sensitive parts of the body like the face and neck to lessen inflammation. People who might not react well to topical corticosteroids or who have reservations about them are frequently prescribed them.

4. Barrier creams and emollients:

Emollients and barrier creams build a barrier that shields the skin from irritation and moisture loss. People with dry and sensitive skin will especially benefit from them.

5. Inhibitors of histamine:

To reduce irritation and encourage better sleep, doctors may prescribe oral antihistamines. There are non-drowsy versions for usage during the day.

6. Therapy using Wet Wraps:

Using moist bandages or garments on moistened skin is known as "wet wrap therapy." Particularly during severe flare-ups, this might help calm and moisturize the skin.

7. Phototherapy: The application of light.

Under controlled circumstances, phototherapy entails exposing the skin to ultraviolet (UV) light. For moderate to severe eczema, it can be a useful treatment, however it is usually applied under medical professionals' supervision.

8. Drugs Used in the System:

Systemic medicines, such as immunosuppressants, biologics, or oral corticosteroids, may be used in situations with severe eczema that do not respond to other therapy. These drugs typically need close observation and are only used in certain circumstances.

9. Determine and Steer Clear of Triggers:

An essential part of managing eczema is recognizing and avoiding irritants that exacerbate symptoms. Making lifestyle changes, such as avoiding particular materials, utilizing hypoallergenic products, and practicing stress management, may be necessary to achieve this.

10. Allergen Immunotherapy (Occasionally):

Allergen immunotherapy may be investigated, under the supervision of an allergist, for those whose eczema is brought on by particular allergens. To desensitize the immune system, the person must be exposed to progressively higher concentrations of the allergen.

Working together with their healthcare providers to create a customized treatment plan is crucial for people with eczema. Depending on the patient's response and evolving circumstances, routine follow-up appointments and modifications to the treatment plan can be required. Long-term management and enhanced quality of life can also be facilitated by upholding healthy lifestyle choices and proper skincare habits.

Skincare and Lifestyle Ideas

The management of eczema and the avoidance of flare-ups are greatly influenced by lifestyle and skincare choices. To promote skin health and reduce triggers, people with eczema can follow certain habits. Important skincare and lifestyle factors for managing eczema include the following:

1. Gentle Skincare Regimen:

Use moisturizers and gentle cleansers without fragrances. Steer clear of abrasive cleansers and soaps that might deplete the skin's natural oils. Select items marked as hypoallergenic and appropriate for delicate skin.

2. Regularly moisturize:

In order to keep the skin barrier intact and avoid dryness, moisturizing is crucial for those who have eczema. After taking a shower, moisturize your skin throughout day, especially in chilly or dry weather.

3. Showers and baths that are too warm:

Instead of using hot water to bathe, use lukewarm water to preserve the skin's natural oils. Keep bath or shower times to ten to fifteen minutes, and use mild cleaning products. Pat dry rather than dabbing with a towel.

4. Don't Scratch:

Scratching can cause skin damage and make eczema symptoms worse. To relieve itching, wear soft cotton gloves at night, trim your nails short, and think about using cold compresses or other distraction strategies.

5. Select Gentle Fabrics:

To reduce skin irritation, dress in breathable, soft materials like cotton. Steer clear of wool and synthetic fabrics as they might lead to irritation and friction.

6. Control your stress:

Eczema flare-ups may be brought on by stress. Exercise stress-reduction methods including yoga, meditation, deep breathing, and other relaxation practices.

7. Recognize and Steer Clear of Triggers

Be mindful of things like specific foods, allergies, or environmental circumstances that can cause flare-ups of eczema. To reduce the possibility of aggravating symptoms, recognize and stay away from certain triggers.

8. Management of Allergens:

Control your exposure if you have someone with eczema brought on by allergies. Using bedding free of allergens, preventing pet dander, and controlling dust mites may all be part of this.

9. Select Hypoallergenic Items:

Whenever possible, choose hypoallergenic skincare, soaps, and detergents. Steer clear of items that include harsh chemicals, colors, or scents since they may irritate skin.

10. Continue Your Nutritious Diet:

Although a specialized diet for eczema does not exist, eating a healthy, well-balanced diet can improve the health of your skin in general. Keep yourself hydrated and think about getting individualized counsel from a certified nutritionist or medical practitioner.

11. Consistent Exercise:

Frequent exercise may aid in stress management and enhance general wellbeing. Pick enjoyable pursuits, and think about working exercise into your schedule.

12. Getting Enough Sleep:

Make sure you receive enough sleep, as insufficient sleep can exacerbate stress and perhaps lead to flare-ups of eczema. For higher-quality sleep, create a regular sleep schedule.

13. Control of the Environment:

Manage environmental elements like temperature and humidity. To keep skin hydrated, stay away from drastic temperature changes and use a humidifier in dry conditions.

14. Protection from the Sun:

To shield the skin from damaging UV radiation, apply sunscreen with a high SPF. Sun protection is essential since sunburn can aggravate eczema symptoms.

Individuals with eczema should work closely with healthcare experts to build a specific skincare routine and lifestyle plan. A higher quality of life and successful eczema management are facilitated by routine follow-up visits and honest discussion with medical specialists.

Coping Mechanisms and Emotional Health

Living with eczema can entail both physical and emotional concerns. Emotional stress may be exacerbated by the obvious symptoms, ongoing itching, and effects on day-to-day functioning. Coping strategies and emphasizing emotional well-being are crucial parts of controlling eczema. Here are coping tactics and recommendations for preserving emotional well-being:

1. Education and Comprehension:

Learn about eczema, its triggers, and effective management strategies. Understanding the disease helps empower individuals to take charge and make informed decisions regarding their care.

2. Help Mechanism:

Build a solid support system by sharing your experiences with family, friends, and healthcare providers. Surround yourself with understanding and caring individuals who can provide emotional support.

3. Open Communication with Healthcare Providers:

Establish open contact with dermatologists or healthcare specialists. Discuss your issues, ask questions, and work jointly to establish a specific treatment plan. Regular follow-up appointments assist address growing needs.

4. Stress Management Techniques:

Practice stress management strategies, such as deep breathing, meditation, mindfulness, or yoga. These approaches can help reduce stress, a known factor for eczema flare-ups.

5. Distraction Techniques:

Engage in activities that distract from itching or discomfort. Reading, listening to music, hobbies, or spending time with loved ones can divert focus and enhance mood.

CHAPTER THREE

6. Psychological Support:

Consider getting psychological support, such as counseling or therapy, to manage the emotional burden of living with eczema. Mental health specialists can provide coping methods and assistance for emotional well-being.

7. Support Groups:

Joining eczema support groups or online forums allows folks to connect with others having similar issues. Sharing experiences, tips, and encouragement can create a sense of connection and understanding.

8. Body Positivity:

Foster a positive body image by concentrating on qualities of yourself beyond eczema. Celebrate achievements, hobbies, and traits that offer delight and contentment.

9. Acceptance and Self-Compassion:

Practice self-acceptance and self-compassion. Accept that eczema is a part of your life, and be kind to yourself. Recognize that controlling eczema is an ongoing process, and setbacks are a typical part of the road.

10. Make sensible goals:

- Set realistic goals and expectations for yourself. Break down larger activities into smaller, doable chunks. Celebrate modest successes and growth.

11. Clothing Choices:

Choose clothing that is comfortable and breathable, minimizing irritation to the skin. Soft, natural textiles like cotton can be more skin-friendly.

12. Set Up a Schedule:

Establishing a steady daily routine can create a sense of stability and predictability. Include specific hours for skincare, relaxation, and self-care.

13. Advocate for Yourself:

Advocate for your needs and communicate openly about your situation with others. Educate friends, colleagues, and instructors about eczema to create understanding and support.

14. Mindful Skincare Practices:

Incorporate skincare routines into your regimen as a form of self-care. Taking care of your skin can be a wonderful and loving experience.

Remember that controlling eczema is a holistic strategy that treats both the physical and mental components of the problem. Prioritizing emotional well-being contributes to a more resilient and optimistic outlook in overcoming the problems connected with eczema.

Children and Eczema

Eczema, or atopic dermatitis, is a common skin condition that can affect children. It often begins in infancy or early childhood and may persist until maturity. Managing eczema in children requires a combination of skincare practices, lifestyle modifications, and, in some circumstances, medication interventions. Here are considerations and solutions for managing eczema in children:

1. Gentle Skincare Practices:

Use moderate, fragrance-free cleansers and moisturizers for your child's skin. Be careful during showering, patting the skin dry instead of rubbing. Keep nails short to reduce skin injury from scratching.

2. Regularly moisturize:

Apply moisturizers to your child's skin periodically, especially after bathing. This helps maintain skin moisture and improves the skin barrier.

3. Select Gentle Fabrics:

Dress your child in soft, breathable fabrics such as cotton. Avoid wool or synthetic items that may cause irritation.

4. Recognize and Steer Clear of Triggers

Pay attention to potential triggers for your child's eczema. These may include certain meals, allergies, or environmental variables. Keep a journal to track probable triggers.

5. Management of Allergens:

If your child has allergies, cooperate with healthcare specialists to monitor and control allergens in the environment. This may involve adopting allergen-proof bedding and minimizing exposure to specific allergens.

6. Establish a Skincare Routine:

Establish a consistent skincare routine for your youngster. Include bathing, moisturizing, and any recommended medications as part of the regimen.

7. Clothing Choices:

Choose attire that is comfortable and non-irritating. Consider utilizing soft cotton clothing to minimize friction and irritation.

8. Be Mindful of Emotional Well-Being:

Children with eczema may have emotional issues owing to itching, discomfort, or the apparent aspect of the disorder. Be supportive, address their worries, and encourage open communication.

9. Avoid Harsh Soaps & Detergents:

Use mild soaps and detergents for your child's laundry to reduce skin irritation. Consider double-rinsing laundry to remove any remaining detergent.

10. Consult Healthcare Professionals:

Work closely with dermatologists or healthcare specialists to check your child's eczema. Regular check-ups and contact with healthcare specialists assist adjust the treatment plan to your child's growing needs.

11. Protection from the Sun:

Protect your child's skin from the sun by wearing sunscreen with a high SPF. Sunburn can aggravate eczema symptoms.

12. Supportive School Environment:

If your child is at school, contact with teachers and school personnel about their eczema. Provide appropriate skincare items and guidance to provide a helpful environment.

13. Emphasize Hydration:

Encourage your youngster to stay hydrated by drinking water throughout the day. Hydration is vital for preserving skin health.

14. Help on an emotional level:

Offer emotional support to your child and educate them about their situation. Help them realize the value of skincare routines and provide reassurance.

15. Seek Professional Guidance for Severe Cases:

In cases of severe eczema that do not respond well to home care, seek expert help. Dermatologists may recommend special medications or therapy customized to your child's requirements.

It's crucial to approach eczema management in children holistically, addressing both physical and mental components. Collaboration with healthcare providers, adhering to a consistent skincare routine, and providing a supportive atmosphere contribute to good eczema management in children.

Pregnancy and Family Planning

Pregnancy and family planning might provide particular challenges for those with eczema. While eczema itself does not normally interfere with conception or pregnancy, several components of controlling eczema may require extra care during this period. Here are some considerations for those with eczema during pregnancy and family planning:

1. Consult with Healthcare Providers:

Before attempting to conceive, check with both your dermatologist and obstetrician/gynecologist. Discuss your plans for pregnancy, and check that your eczema management strategy is acceptable for this period.

2. Evaluation of Medication:

Review any drugs used to control eczema with healthcare providers. Some drugs may need changes or temporary discontinuance during pregnancy, as certain compounds may represent potential dangers to the growing fetus.

3. Pregnancy-Safe Skincare:

Choose pregnancy-safe skincare products. Some elements typically found in skincare products may be best avoided during pregnancy. Consult with healthcare providers or dermatologists for assistance on safe products.

4. Hydration and Moisturization:

Maintain appropriate hydration and moisturization to support skin health during pregnancy. Pregnancy-related hormonal changes can influence skin issues, and keeping the skin well-hydrated may help decrease symptoms.

5. Emphasize Stress Management:

Pregnancy may be a stressful time, and stress is a known trigger for eczema flare-ups. Emphasize stress management skills such as relaxation, meditation, and mindfulness.

6. Allergy Considerations:

Pregnancy can occasionally lead to changes in allergies and sensitivities. Pay attention to any new triggers or exacerbation of eczema symptoms and discuss them with healthcare specialists.

7. Clothing Choices:

Choose soft, breathable fabrics for clothing, as the skin may be more sensitive during pregnancy. Comfortable clothing can assist prevent friction and irritation.

8. Protection from the Sun:

If spending time outdoors, use pregnancy-safe sunscreen with a high SPF to protect the skin from the sun. solar protection is necessary, as pregnancy-related changes might make the skin more susceptible to solar harm.

9. Honest Communication:

Maintain open contact with healthcare providers about any changes in eczema symptoms, skin condition, or overall well-being throughout pregnancy. Regular check-ups can help monitor both maternal and fetal health.

10. Postpartum Care:

After childbirth, continue to focus skincare and well-being. Hormonal changes postpartum may affect eczema symptoms, so be sensitive to any changes and seek help from healthcare specialists.

11. Considering Breastfeeding:

If breastfeeding, check healthcare practitioners about the safety of any drugs used for eczema. Many topical therapies are generally considered safe during nursing, although expert assistance is required.

12. Family Planning with Eczema Management in Mind:

If family planning entails spacing pregnancies, consider the influence of hormonal shifts and stress on eczema symptoms. Plan for enough support throughout these periods.

Every pregnancy is unique, and individual circumstances differ. The goal is to engage with healthcare experts, maintain open communication, and adjust eczema management options to the personal needs and preferences of the individual during pregnancy and family planning.

Alternative Therapies and Home Remedies

While established medical treatments are often suggested for controlling eczema, some individuals may investigate alternative therapies and home remedies to complement their overall care. It's crucial to highlight that alternative therapies should be discussed with healthcare practitioners, and their effectiveness may vary from person to person. Here are some alternative therapies and home remedies that patients with eczema may consider:

1. Coconut Oil:

Applying virgin coconut oil to the afflicted areas may help hydrate the skin and relieve inflammation. Coconut oil has antibacterial qualities and can be a natural alternative to conventional moisturizers.

2. Oatmeal Baths:

Taking oatmeal baths may provide relief from itching and inflammation. Colloidal oatmeal can be added to warm bathwater to soothe the skin. After showering, pat the skin dry and apply a moisturizer.

3. Honey:

Applying raw honey to eczema spots may have antibacterial and anti-inflammatory qualities. Ensure the honey is pure and test on a small patch of skin to check for any unwanted effects.

4. Aloe Vera:

Aloe vera gel, produced from the leaves of the aloe plant, is known for its soothing effects. Applying aloe vera gel to eczema-affected areas may help reduce redness and irritation.

5. Evening Primrose Oil:

Evening primrose oil, taken orally or used topically, is rich in gamma-linolenic acid (GLA), which may have anti-inflammatory properties.

Consult with healthcare providers before utilizing supplements.

6. Probiotics:

Probiotics, either through supplements or probiotic-rich foods, may help balance gut flora and perhaps alter immunological responses. Some patients with eczema may find probiotics beneficial, but further research is needed.

7. Chamomile:

Chamomile, whether in the form of chamomile tea or chamomile extract, is known for its anti-inflammatory and relaxing effects. It can be administered topically or taken as a tea.

8. Calendula:

Calendula cream or ointment, derived from the marigold plant, is claimed to have anti-inflammatory qualities. It may be administered to eczema-prone areas.

9. Sunflower Seed Oil:

Sunflower seed oil is a natural emollient that may assist enhance skin moisture. Applying sunflower seed oil to the skin can aid to moisturization.

10. Methods for Lowering Stress:

Practices such as meditation, deep breathing exercises, and yoga may help manage stress, a known trigger for eczema flare-ups.

11. Acupuncture:

Acupuncture involves the insertion of tiny needles into precise spots on the body. Some patients with eczema may find acupuncture useful, but its efficacy varies.

12. Wet Wrap Therapy with Diluted Bleach:

Wet wrap therapy includes administering a diluted bleach solution to the skin before wrapping it in wet bandages. This procedure may be recommended by healthcare providers in specific instances.

13. Tea Tree Oil (Caution):

Tea tree oil, when diluted, may have antibacterial effects. However, it might be annoying to some individuals, and it should be used gently.

Perform a patch test and speak with healthcare providers before use.

It's vital to approach alternative therapies with caution and to check with healthcare specialists before trying new treatments, especially when it comes to dietary supplements or topical applications. While some individuals may find relief from certain alternative therapies, the major focus should be on evidence-based medical treatments and a thorough eczema care strategy.

Conclusion

In conclusion, eczema, or atopic dermatitis, is a widespread chronic skin disorder marked by inflammation, itching, and recurring flare-ups.

While the actual origin of eczema is complex and diverse, it involves a combination of genetic, immunologic, and environmental factors. Eczema can greatly damage the quality of life of affected persons, resulting to discomfort, sleep difficulties, and emotional challenges.

The management of eczema often entails a complex approach, including skincare practices, lifestyle adjustments, and, in some situations, medication therapies. Moisturization, avoidance of triggers, and the use of topical corticosteroids or other recommended drugs are critical components of treatment. In recent years, improvements in research have led to the introduction of targeted medicines, including biologics, topical JAK inhibitors, and a clearer understanding of the role of the skin microbiota.

Individuals with eczema should work closely with healthcare specialists to build tailored treatment strategies, addressing the particular elements of their condition. It's crucial to address not only the physical symptoms but also the emotional well-being of those with eczema, as stress and mental health can effect the illness.

As research continues to advance, there is optimism for the development of more tailored and effective treatments for eczema. Digital health solutions, patient-centric approaches, and ongoing research to understand the underlying mechanisms of the condition lead to a more complete and tailored approach to eczema therapy.

While eczema may provide challenges, especially during flare-ups, with careful care and commitment to treatment plans, many individuals can effectively control their symptoms and enjoy satisfying lives. Staying educated about the latest research and getting assistance from healthcare professionals and the eczema community helps empower individuals to negotiate the complexity of this chronic skin condition.

THE END